Coping with the long term effect
A true life story

Part 7
Mental challenge on ovarian cancer
Educating the future generation

Conclusion
Reference

Introduction

One disease that affects women is ovarian cancer. This type of cancer occurs when abnormalities in certain ovarian cells develop and multiply uncontrollably. resulting in tumors The ovaries are the female reproductive organs that produce eggs. Most ovarian cancers occur after age 60, with approximately 90% of cases occurring after age 40. The cells that line the cavities and surfaces of the body are called epithelial cells. And this is where the most common type of ovarian cancer begins. These cancers can develop in the epithelial cells of the ovaries. But from research Most ovarian cancers begin in the epithelial cells at the fimbria, or the edges at the ends of the fallopian tubes and ovaries where cancer cells go. Cancer can also develop in the epithelial cells that make up the peritoneum. This type of cancer is known as peritoneal cancer. The origins, symptoms, progression, and treatment of peritoneal cancer are similar. The ovaries are frequently affected by peritoneal cancer. It can still occur even after the ovaries are removed. Cancers that start in the ovaries, fallopian tubes, and peritoneum are often difficult to distinguish. This is because they are very similar and can spread quickly from one structure to another. These cancers are so closely related that they are often considered together by experts. In about 10% of cases, ovarian cancer originates in granulosa cells, which are ovarian cells that produce hormones. or reproductive cells, which are the origins of ovarian cells And there are generally no symptoms in the early stages of ovarian

PREFACE

There are times when we have to face difficult realities. Speak up and act decisively to protect the future of our ever-changing world. protracted silence Whether it is due to fear, complacency, or ignorance. hinder progress This is especially true when it comes to the most important issues of our time, such as social injustice, human rights, climate change. and health crisis These are not remote problems. They affect everyone and help shape the world for generations to come.

The choices we make today will determine the legacy we leave behind at this turning point in history. Speaking up is just one aspect of breaking the silence. Others include listening, recognizing voices that have been suppressed for too long. and determination to proceed Call for courage sympathy and a sense of duty to the people who took our world from us.

In addition to the need to protect the environment, health and peace, Protecting the lives of future generations Going is also important. It is an investment in humanity's potential. It is about giving our children, grandchildren and great-grandchildren the opportunity to live a just, healthy and sustainable life. Only by working together can we achieve this goal. whether it is anti-inequality Stopping climate change Guaranteeing universal access to health care and aiming for a society where all voices are respected and heard.

This identification serves as a rallying cry. It forces us to transcend the realm of silence. Heed urgent requests for help. And choices must be made now that will not only save lives, but also save lives. But it also helps build a better future. We are doing this work not only for ourselves but for generations to come. It is time to speak up, take action, and protect the future to ensure that we leave behind a world where justice, health, and hope can blossom.

Content

Part 1
What is cancer
What is ovaries
What is ovarian cancer
Type of ovarian cancer

Part 2
Challenge of ovarian cancer
From patient perspective
From doctor perspective
Reason for late diagnosed
The key to early diagnosis

Part 3
Advocating for early detection
Important of self awareness
Detecting overian cancer early important note for woman

Part 4
Why ovarian cancer need more attention
Lack of public awareness on ovarian cancer
How you can help family and friends

Part 5
Understanding your body
Knowing your family history

Part 6
Life after ovarian cancer
Coping with short term effect

cancer compared to epithelial cells- Back pain, bloating, feeling full immediately after eating. Vaginal bleeding during or after menstruation Changes in bowel or urinary behavior Pain or heaviness in the pelvis or lower abdomen These are some of the symptoms that can be detected when cancer has spread. Just because a woman has one or more of these symptoms does not mean she has ovarian cancer. Sometimes a malignant tumor can attack nearby tissue and spread to other parts. of the body Cancerous tumors usually occur in the abdominal cavity or on the outside of organs near the bladder or colon. If ovarian cancer has spread Metastatic cancer is a tumor that starts in one place and spreads to other parts of the body. Some types of ovarian cancer run in families. These cancers involve inherited gene mutations and are characterized by genetic inheritance. Compared to non-hereditary (sporadic) cases, hereditary ovarian cancer tends to be discovered at a young age. Ovarian cancer kills more women in the United States each year than any other gynecological cancer. Can be difficult to maintain Because it is often detected late But it has a high five-year survival rate when it is identified and treated early.

Part 1

What is cancer?

Cancer is a disease caused by cells. Tissues and organs are made up of cells, which are the basic building blocks of the body. The body continually produces new cells to support growth. Repair damaged tissue and promote wound healing Normally, cells divide and die systematically. Each new cell replaces the lost cell. However, sometimes the cell becomes abnormal and continues to multiply. Cancer can develop from these abnormally shaped cells. In solid cancers, such as ovarian cancer, abnormally shaped cells form a lump or lump called a tumor. Abnormally shaped cells accumulate in the blood in some cancers, such as leukemia. Uncontrolled cell proliferation This results in the development of malignant tumors or the formation of abnormal cells in the tissue resembling blood. It is considered a hallmark of cancer. This is a complex disease with many facets. Cancer develops at the cellular level when regulatory processes control cell division. Growth and death are disrupted, the genetic material (DNA) that encodes instructions for cell function. Including the process of regulating the cell cycle. cell death Cell death (programmed cell death) and DNA repair tightly control these mechanisms.

Cell proliferation in healthy tissue is tightly regulated to meet the body's physiological needs, such as tissue growth, wound healing, and replacement of damaged cells. And this regulation includes the phosphoinositide 3-kinase (PI3K)/Akt pathway and the mitogen-activated protein kinase (MAPK) pathway, which regulate the cell cycle. Several signaling pathways involve G1 (cell growth), S (DNA replication), G2 (mitosis formation) and M (mitosis or cell division) phases. that make up the cell cycle At different stages of the cycle, the integrity of the DNA is assessed and if it is damaged. Repair mechanisms are stimulated. To prevent the spread of damaged or potentially cancerous cells. Cells are ordered to undergo apoptosis if the damage is irreversible.

However, these regulatory mechanisms are circumvented or disrupted in cancer cells. Uncontrolled cell division can result from mutations in genes that control the cell cycle, such as tumor suppressor genes and proto-oncogenes. When mutated Proto-oncogenes become oncogenes that promote cell division. While inactive tumor suppressor genes such as p53 are unable to prevent abnormal cell division, additional mutations can develop that help create carcinogens. This is aggravated by defects in DNA repair mechanisms, as in Lynch syndrome... observed in hereditary cancer syndromes.

These abnormal cells often develop into localized lumps or lumps in solid tumors, such as ovarian cancer, which can infiltrate adjacent tissue and may spread (spread) to other parts of the body through the lymph or lymphatic fluid. circulatory system Tumor cells, stromal cells, immune cells extracellular matrix Composition and microenvironment of tumors...pattern which is necessary for tumor growth Normal cell function, such as creating new blood vessels The formation of new blood vessels is usually eliminated by the tumor that supplies it with oxygen and Nutrients to stimulate growth.

 Instead it develops into a solid tumor. Malformed cells proliferate in the bone marrow and blood in blood cancers such as leukemia. A red blood cell disorder that produces different types of blood cells. It is a factor in leukemia. These malformed cells replace Healthy red blood cells in leukemia By disrupting oxygen transport in blood clotting and immune response. Normal cell signaling pathways that control immune surveillance may be disrupted by cancer. This allows tumors to evade recognition and destruction by the immune system. Several strategies exist for achieving immune evasion, such as the expression of immune checkpoint molecules such as PD-L1, which suppress the immune response. It is used to identify and fight cancer cells. Restoring the body's immune response is the goal of immunotherapy. which is a branch that is expanding rapidly of cancer treatment...

In addition, various environmental, lifestyle and epigenetic factors It also contributes to the development of cancer. It's not just genetic diseases: Radiation, cigarette smoke, and certain viruses are examples of environmental factors that can cause DNA mutations that trigger cancer. Histone modifications and DNA methylation are examples of epigenetic modifications that can alter gene expression without changing the underlying genetic code. which promotes the production of carcinogenic substances.

Targeted therapy and personalized medicine It attempts to inhibit specific molecular drivers of cancer to reduce harm to normal cells. It was developed as a result of a better understanding of the complex molecular mechanisms that cause cancer. More research is needed to establish

In summary, cancer is a disorder of normal cellular functions such as immune surveillance, DNA repair, and cell death. and cell cycle control Molecular complexity requires a comprehensive understanding of pathology. cell biology and genetics to guide cancer prevention treatment plans. The cellular and molecular bases of cancer are becoming better understood. Due to continuous advancements in cancer research This opens the door to more specific and effective treatments…

What is ovaries

Together with the uterus, cervix (uterus), uterus (uterus), vagina (vagina), and vulva (external genitalia), the ovaries are components of the female reproductive system. The ovaries are an important component of the female reproductive system as they produce eggs. or eggs and hormones that control various aspects of reproductive health Its side is located in the pelvic cavity, which is an important part of the overall reproductive system function. Fertility and Hormone Balance

The process of producing eggs is central to ovarian function and is also known as ovulation. The number of immature eggs in the ovaries is limited at birth. and will gradually decrease throughout a woman's life A number of follicles grow each menstrual cycle, however, usually only one follicle is strong enough to release a mature egg at ovulation. Although multiple eggs may sometimes ripen in cases of multiple oocytes. But this process guarantees that only one egg will be ready for fertilization...

As an endocrine gland The ovaries also produce progesterone and estrogen. which is necessary for regulating the menstrual cycle In addition to affecting the thickness of the uterine lining during pregnancy, Estrogen also plays a role in the development of secondary.
Sexual characteristics such as breast development and body hair growth after ovulation Progesterone is produced to maintain the uterine lining for a potential pregnancy and help implant the fertilized egg. The ovarian cycle is controlled by gonadotropins, such as follicle-stimulating hormone (FSH) and luteinizing hormone (LH), which interact with each other Of these hormones and the hypothalamus are secreted by the pituitary gland.

The uterus, cervix, uterus, vagina, and vulva are all components of the larger female reproductive system. The ovary is only one component. And each element has a specific function in pregnancy, birth, and reproduction. The fallopian tubes are often the site of fertilization. This is especially important for capturing the egg released during ovulation. The fertilized egg is transported to the uterus for development and implantation. Menstruation causes the lining of the uterus to thicken in the absence of fertilization.

The uterus is located at the lower end of the uterus. Helps menstrual blood and semen pass easily during intercourse. In addition to the production of mucus in the uterus which can promote or hinder sperm movement It depends on the regularity throughout the menstrual cycle.

 The external genitals or vagina act as a barrier to protect the internal reproductive organs, the vagina, including the labia, clitoris, and vaginal invaginations. It also contributes to sexual happiness. Each component of the reproductive system is interconnected and works together to maintain optimal fertility and reproductive health.

Diagnosing and treating reproductive health problems requires an understanding of the complex relationships between the ovaries and other organs. of the reproductive system One or more of these organs can become dysfunctional in conditions such as infertility, ovarian cancer, and polycystic ovary syndrome (PCOS) due to the system's complex hormonal regulation. Fertility and general health Maintenance of ovarian health is therefore important for fertility and general reproductive well-being..

Now we dive into the bigger question what ovarian cancer

Any growth of malignancy That begins in a woman's ovaries, which are the organs that produce eggs. It's called ovarian cancer. In the early stages, there are usually no symptoms, although vaginal bleeding, pain, or pressure in the lower abdomen may occur. Ovarian cancer is a type of cancer that begins in the ovaries, which are the reproductive organs that produce eggs, progesterone, estrogen, and other hormones. In the pelvic area of women The ovaries are located on one side of the uterus. The term "ovarian cancer" refers to several types of cancer, including stromal, germ cell, and germ cell cancer. and epithelial tumors that can develop from cells in the ovaries. The biological behavior of each species is different. Epithelial ovarian cancer is the most common type.

This is because they do not show clear symptoms until they have spread to other areas. of the abdomen or pelvis Ovarian cancer is therefore often not diagnosed in its early stages. and when symptoms appear Cancer can also be obscure and confused with less serious diseases. Mild abdominal pain, bloating, and a feeling of fullness or fullness in the abdomen are examples of early symptoms. This discomfort is sometimes confused with bloating for less serious causes, such as digestive problems.

The severity of symptoms increases as the disease progresses. People often report periodic or chronic pain in the lower abdomen or pelvic area. This pain can be caused by tumor growth. which puts pressure on nearby organs or tissues and makes you feel uncomfortable If the tumor is large enough It may affect bowel or bladder function. This can lead to constipation. The stool is void. Or urinate frequently.

Vaginal bleeding is another important symptom that can indicate ovarian cancer, especially after menopause. Although vaginal bleeding is often related to hormonal imbalance or cervical cancer, But it may also be a warning sign of ovarian cancer in postmenopausal women. Menstruation that lasts longer than normal or irregular cycles can indicate a developing problem in premenopausal women.

Early detection of ovarian cancer is challenging because of the unprecedented sensitivity of these symptoms. The disease is often discovered after it has spread. This makes treatment complex. For this reason, prompt medical advice and awareness of mild symptoms are essential for timely diagnosis and a good outcome. A number of genetic, molecular and cellular changes can cause abnormal cells in the ovaries to grow and spread out of control, such as developing ovarian cancer. This is because ovarian hormones are responsible for producing eggs. Routine surgical intervention can cause cancer. This process begins when normal ovarian cells accumulate genetic mutations that change their specific behavior and lead to uncontrolled cell division. Many genes, including cancer-causing genes, that controls DNA repair and cell growth and tumor suppressor genes There is a risk of these mutations. For example, the risk of ovarian cancer is greatly increased by mutations in the BRCA1 or BRCA2 genes, which normally help repair damaged DNA. Cells are more likely to develop additional genetic changes that cause Uncontrolled growth occurs when these genes are mutated..

These mutations disrupt the normal cell cycle at the molecular level. Prevents damaged cells from apoptosis. or programmed cell death These damaged cells do not die. Instead, it divides and grows into a tumor. even from other cells, such as reproductive cells (which produce eggs) or stromal cells Ovarian cancer usually begins in the epithelial cells that line the surface of the ovary. These altered cells begin to multiply in epithelial ovarian cancer. by change The natural structure of the ovaries is being created.

.

Changes in the surrounding environment support tumor growth. Tumor progression is significantly affected by the ovarian tumor microenvironment (TME), which includes the extracellular matrix. immune cells and blood vessels. Tumor cancer cells can release many chemicals. Includes cytokines and growth factors that promote angiogenesis. (creation of new blood, blood vessels) tumors, nutrients and oxygen are supplied This vasodilation helps tumors grow and invade surrounding tissue.

As ovarian cancer progresses The cancer will begin to spread outside the ovaries. Invasion of adjacent pelvic cavity structures, such as the cervix, bowel, or uterus, may be the first step in this spread. But when the tumor spreads Cancer cells may also be released into the abdominal cavity lining the abdominal cavity. Then it spread to other parts. of the abdomen and pelvis to form secondary tumors A key component in the development of ovarian cancer is metastasis. Cancer cells also have the ability to travel through the bloodstream or lymphatic system to distant organs, such as the liver or lungs, where they can spread. Can develop into a secondary tumor.

One of his problems is his ability to avoid early detection of ovarian cancer. In the initial stage Ovarian cancer often presents with very vague symptoms, such as mild abdominal discomfort or bloating. or not showing symptoms It is easy to confuse these symptoms with less serious illnesses. When symptoms are more severe, such as vaginal bleeding or pelvic pain Cancer may also spread to other areas. Makes treatment difficult...

In addition, as time passes Ovarian cancer cells can also become resistant to treatment. Genetic changes in tumor cells that allow them to tolerate chemotherapy or targeted therapy are often the cause of this resistance. For example, efflux pumps, which remove chemotherapy drugs from cells before they have an effect. that causes damage It is more effective in ovarian cancer cells. Resistance can arise from other mechanisms, such as changes in DNA repair pathways or tumor genetics.

In summary, ovarian cancer occurs due to the slow accumulation of genetic mutations. which disrupts normal cellular processes This results in uncontrolled cell proliferation and tumor development. Cancer complications increase with resistance to treatment. And it is also difficult to detect early on. A better understanding of the genetic and molecular mechanisms underlying the development of ovarian cancer is needed to improve early diagnosis and treatment approaches...

The different type of ovarian cancer and Symptoms

Many types of cancer that begin in the ovaries are included in the general term "ovarian cancer." The cells in which they develop and their biology separate these different types. Germ cell tumor Stromal tumor and epithelial ovarian cancer are the three main forms of ovarian cancer. This is because these types vary in development. Prognosis and treatment plan Therefore, it is very important to understand these things. Each type is described in detail below. With advice on management and treatment by medical experts.:

1. Epithelial Ovarian Cancer

About 90% of all ovarian cancers are epithelial. Therefore, it is the most common type of cancer. The epithelial cells covering the surface of the ovary are the source. Histopathological characteristics of tumor cells are used to classify this type of cancer into additional subtypes. Aggressive cancer, which can be high-grade or low-grade, is the most common subtype. Mucosal cancer Endometriosis and clear cell carcinoma as an additional subtype.

Development and Risk Factors:

Because epithelial ovarian cancer often causes no symptoms in its early stages, it often takes years to develop and be discovered in an advanced stage. Especially after menopause. which increases the risk of developing epithelial ovarian cancer. Family history of breast or ovarian cancer Genetic mutations, such as in the BRCA1 and BRCA2 genes, also increase the risk.

Symptoms:

bloating pelvic pain Feeling full quickly And changes in bowel habits are often symptoms in the early stages and are often not obvious. Changes in your menstrual cycle or more severe pain can be a result of fibroid growth. Vaginal bleeding is another alarming symptom. Especially after menopause

Medical Advice and Treatment:

Early detection considered important But this may be difficult because the symptoms are mild. Surgery and chemotherapy are commonly used to treat patients with epithelial ovarian cancer. Surgical methods to achieve optimal removal Neoplasia (removal of as much tumor tissue as possible) usually involves the removal of the uterus, fallopian tubes, ovaries, and surrounding lymph nodes. Often used with taxanes (such as paclitaxel), platinum-based chemotherapy includes carboplatin and cisplatin. in a specific situation Targeted treatments such as anti-angiogenic drugs may also be used. or PARP inhibitors (for patients with BRCA mutations). Immunotherapy may also be an option for patients with advanced disease.

2. Germ Cell Tumors

Only 5% of ovarian cancers are germ cell tumors. making it much less common Cells in the ovaries that normally develop into eggs cause these tumors. Although germ cell tumors can develop at any age, But young women and teenage girls are most often diagnosed. Most of these tumors are benign. But some types can be malignant, such as tumors in the sinuses of the skin. and disgerminoma which is the most common type of malignant germ cell tumor...

Development and Risk Factors:

Ovarian oocytes cause germ cell tumors. Although in many cases the cause is unknown. But genetic factors, such as mutations in cancer suppressor genes or a family history of cancer May increase risk Germ cell tumors often appear before epithelial ovarian cancer.

Symptoms:

Some possible symptoms include abdominal pain, bloating, or a noticeable lump in the abdomen. Hormonal imbalances caused by fibroids can sometimes result in symptoms such as irregular periods. Too much hair growing or breast tissue changes...

Medical Advice and Treatment:

When detected early Germ cell tumors are often easier to treat than epithelial and ovarian cancers. The main treatment is surgery. The aim is to remove the tumor and leave the ovary intact, if possible. Especially in young women who want to preserve their fertility. This is especially true in cases of advanced or metastatic disease. Surgery and chemotherapy are often combined. Bleomycin, etoposide, cisplatin, or BEP chemotherapy are commonly used to treat malignant germ cell tumors. The prognosis is usually favorable. Especially for tumors in the early stages.

3. Stromal Tumors

The connective tissue cells (stroma) that support the ovaries and produce hormones such as progesterone and estrogen are the source of stromal tumors. These tumors account for 5-7% of ovarian cancer cases. They release hormones. Causes symptoms related to hormonal imbalance and may not be severe or even fatal.

Types of Stromal Tumors:

Granulose cell tumor and granulomatous cell tumor Sertoli-Leydig It is the main form of stromal tumor. The most common type of granulomatous cell tumor usually produces estrogen. This may result in abnormal bleeding or other symptoms. of excessive hormones, Sertoli-Leydig cells... Tumors can also produce testosterone and, less frequently, cause signs of masculinity, such as increased body hair or a darker tone.

Development and Risk Factors:

Granulosa cell tumors are most often diagnosed in postmenopausal women. While stromal cell tumors commonly affect women of all ages, The development of these tumors is usually associated with a mutation in the FOXL2 gene. Especially granulosa cell tumors. May be influenced by hormonal factors.

Symptoms:

This is due to the production of estrogen. Patients with granulosa cell tumors may have abnormal uterine bleeding. Including menopausal bleeding. Other than a pelvic mass or abdominal pain Increased facial hair or a deep voice are examples of signs of masculinization that can result from melanoma. Sertoli-Leydig

Medical Advice and Treatment:

Treatment for stromal tumors usually involves surgical removal of the tumor. Frequent removal of the uterus and ovaries. Especially in the case of malignant tumors. And the prognosis is often favorable for patients with early-stage disease. For tumors that have spread or recurred Chemotherapy and radiation may be considered. Hormone therapy may be used in certain situations. This is especially true if the tumor secretes hormones.

In summary, several types of tumors fall under the umbrella of ovarian cancer. Each type has unique clinical characteristics, risk factors, and treatment. The most common type of ovarian cancer, epithelial, often appears late and requires aggressive chemotherapy and surgery. Younger women are more likely to develop germ cell tumors. This is generally easier to treat with surgery and chemotherapy. Although stromal tumors are rare, But it can cause hormonal symptoms. need to have surgery and if detected early will have a good prognosis

Women should be aware of their own bodies. Seek medical help if symptoms such as bloating and pelvic pain persist. abnormal bleeding People with a family history of breast or ovarian cancer may be advised to undergo genetic counseling and testing. Because identifying high-risk individuals leads to to early detection of ovarian cancer and preventive surgery or preventive measures such as surveillance. Currently, there is no routine screening for ovarian cancer. But regular gynecological exams, especially for known risk factors, can help detect ovarian abnormalities in the first place…

Part 2

The challenge of diagnosis

Ovarian cancer is often overlooked by women and medical professionals. This is due to the nature of the disease, its symptoms and the difficulty in early diagnosis.

From the Patient's Perspective:

It is true that the symptoms of ovarian cancer are often vague and non-specific. Considered one of the biggest barriers to early detection, minor symptoms such as bloating, abdominal pain, and changes in bowel or urination can cause discomfort in women. These are symptoms that can be easily attributed to less serious and more widespread conditions such as gas, indigestion, irritable bowel syndrome. or menstruation is irregular Women don't immediately associate their symptoms with something as serious as cancer because it's common.

Moreover, even if it happens These symptoms are usually not severe enough to compel a woman to see a doctor immediately. Fear and rejection are two psychological factors that can cause delays in seeking help. Avoiding the topic altogether may be a result of fear of ovarian cancer. This is a condition that is notoriously difficult to treat in advanced stages. Women with a family history of cancer also feel resigned or dying. This causes them to stop going to the doctor because they believe they have There is nothing they can do if they have cancer, which is possible.

Additionally, ovarian cancer is not widely known. Especially in younger women Ovarian cancer is not as well known as breast cancer. It is actively promoted in public health campaigns and awareness initiatives. It is possible that many women are not aware that their symptoms could be symptoms of ovarian cancer. This knowledge gap is aggravated by the lack of standardized ovarian cancer screening techniques. It's not like a mammogram for breast cancer...

In addition, elderly women, especially postmenopausal women, are often affected by ovarian cancer. Symptoms at this point include bloating or abnormal bleeding. They may be misdiagnosed as a result of old age or other normal conditions. related to aging, such as gastrointestinal disorders or hormonal changes Many women this age don't immediately think they have cancer before talking. See a doctor about their concerns. They are waiting

From the Healthcare Professional's Perspective:

Ovarian cancer can be difficult for medical professionals to identify early on. This is because symptoms are often vague and subtle. There is no standard screening test for ovarian cancer. Unlike cancers such as breast cancer, which can be identified with standard screening techniques such as mammograms, early detection of ovarian cancer is more difficult due to the lack of reliable, non-invasive techniques.

Doctors often treat conditions such as abnormal bowel movements. Pelvic pain and bloating, non-serious gynecological problems such as gastrointestinal disorders urinary tract infection Uterine tumors or cysts in the ovaries It can cause these symptoms. Doctors may prefer these more common diagnoses. Because ovarian cancer is relatively uncommon compared to these other diseases, ovarian cancer is more likely to go away with symptoms such as: Other conditions Many of these can make early identification difficult.

Additionally, many healthcare workers can be under significant time pressure. This is especially true in primary care settings where doctors may be more focused on treating urgent problems or managing chronic conditions. Ovarian cancer symptoms do not appear. Unlike other cancer symptoms, such as lumps or skin changes, these "red flags" are specific and temporary. When there is a history of general disease Doctors can focus more on timely diagnosis or simple diagnosis.

This is due to the complexity of existing tests and the possibility of false positive results. Doctors are sometimes reluctant to pursue ovarian cancer that is too aggressive for diagnosis. Although blood tests such as the CA-125 marker or imaging modalities such as CT and ultrasound scans can be helpful, It is not a reliable method for diagnosing ovarian cancer, for example. Elevated CA-125 levels can occur in many situations. This includes endometriosis, pregnancy, or benign ovarian cysts. In the same way Intravenous ultrasound can identify ovarian abnormalities. But it cannot be determined whether it is benign or not. As a result, doctors may be reluctant to order additional tests right away. Especially when they calculate the significant mental costs. and the financial and physical costs associated with invasive diagnostic procedures...

In addition, the low prevalence of ovarian cancer in the general population may help reduce the skepticism of doctors treating patients at average risk for the disease. Ovarian cancer is considered a more likely diagnosis only if the patient presents with more severe symptoms, such as persistent abdominal pain or irregular bleeding, with good results.

Combined Challenges:

Ovarian cancer can go undetected or misdiagnosed in its early stages due to factors such as minor symptoms and lack of awareness. Lack of reliable screening methods High incidence of other common conditions

Although doctors can use a variety of diagnostic methods, This includes imaging studies, blood tests, and sometimes exploratory surgery. It can be difficult to recognize that symptoms that are often viewed as benign may actually be signs of a serious condition. which is getting more and more difficult This is due to a lack of knowledge about early warning signs of the disease among the general public and medical professionals.

However, the importance of educating patients and health care professionals about ovarian cancer is important. symptoms of cancer and the need for early intervention. It has been recently emphasized that health care providers should be aware of the differential diagnosis of ovarian cancer when a woman has persistent pregnancy symptoms. This is especially important if there is It's family history. To increase the chance of early detection and effective treatment The aim should be to raise awareness and promote early screening and counseling..

.Here are the reasons why its been diagnosed at late stage

Early detection of ovarian cancer It is very challenging. And the disease often becomes more severe once it's detected. Several factors both from the perspective of the patient and the health care provider. It plays an important role in this delayed diagnosis. Abdominal or pelvic pain, bloating, feeling full quickly. Difficulty eating and urinary problems These are all vague and non-specific symptoms of ovarian cancer. This often mimics other symptoms. Many others are much less serious, 1999, which makes treatment much more difficult.

Lack of clear and predictable symptoms is the main reason for delayed diagnosis. In its early stages, ovarian cancer may have mild or uncomfortable symptoms that are ignored or mistaken for a less serious and more common disease. Bloating, abdominal pain, and changes in stool. or the common symptoms of digestive problems such as gas, constipation or irritable bowel syndrome (IBS) that women may experience. Because of this, women never consider the possibility of ovarian cancer. The onset of symptoms may be mild and gradual. Therefore, it is not serious or urgent enough to see a doctor immediately. Many women, especially those without a family history of ovarian cancer These symptoms are often not seen as indicators of a serious health problem. Blame it on hormonal fluctuations, stress, or dietary changes instead...

Women and medical professionals often overlook cancer in favor of more common cancers. At least it can be diagnosed. Even if symptoms persist This is due to less obvious or serious symptoms such as indigestion, the effects of aging. Hormonal changes during menstruation It can easily be blamed for all the pelvic discomfort or bloating and then peeing. Urgency or frequent urination can be confused with pelvic floor dysfunction or a urinary tract infection. This is a much more common condition. These overlapping symptoms do not immediately increase the possibility of ovarian cancer. and often results in incorrect diagnosis. Delaying proper treatment...

Early detection It is further complicated by the deep anatomical location of the ovaries. This is because the ovaries are hidden deep in the pelvic cavity. A tumor may not appear as a mass or mass during standard examinations. This is different from breast cancer, which can be identified through a mammogram or self-exam. Ovarian tumors often develop without any outwardly noticeable symptoms. Your doctor can also look for symptoms during a regular pelvic exam. Especially if there is no visible lump until the tumor is large enough to affect nearby organs without causing obvious problems. When that time comes The cancer may have spread outside the ovaries. and often results in worsening symptoms

Early detection of ovarian cancer poses additional problems for the medical community. There is currently no routine screening for ovarian cancer. It's not like other types of cancer. Although it can be used to detect ovarian abnormalities, tests such as the CA-125 blood test and pelvic ultrasound are not definitive diagnostic methods. CA-125 levels can also be increased in many other conditions, such as: Benign ovarian cysts Fibroids and menstrual cycle Pelvic ultrasound shows abnormalities But it cannot be determined whether it is benign or not. These limitations may make doctors reluctant to immediately order further testing. This is especially true if the patient does not have serious risk factors for ovarian cancer. or if the symptoms are not severe And even diseases like ovarian cancer are becoming more prevalent. This allows medical professionals to prioritize other diagnoses than cancer...

The mental illness that ovarian cancer causes to patients and healthcare professionals is another contributing factor. This is because ovarian cancer has a poor prognosis. Especially if it is detected at an advanced stage. The possibility of cancer is therefore frightening. From this fact Patients and doctors may experience emotional barriers. Women expressed reluctance to consider cancer as a possible cause. Because it may be scary or unexpected. They postpone seeking medical help or keep their concerns to themselves until symptoms become unbearable, fearing the worst but hoping for a less serious explanation. But medical professionals are reluctant to diagnose ovarian cancer early. Because they don't want to worry about taking care of patients. With not many serious diseases Ovarian cancer research has often progressed more slowly as a result of a reluctance to raise the topic of cancer and a lack of reliable diagnostic indicators.

Doctors focus on more common symptoms than ovarian cancer. This is because many women undergoing treatment must first be diagnosed with the disease. Ovarian cancer is only considered if symptoms persist or worsen. By that time the disease will have spread a lot. At this point the peritoneum lymph nodes or other organs The abdominal cavity can be affected by cancer. This makes treatment more difficult and treatment less successful. At this stage the prognosis is usually not good. Because when ovarian cancer spreads outside the ovary, it usually responds less than treatment.

Finally, the general public and some health care facilities are often not aware of ovarian cancer. Ovarian cancer does not receive the same attention as breast cancer. This is despite the fact that ovarian cancer is the subject of widespread awareness campaigns. Gaps in public awareness prevent many women from understanding the significance of their symptoms or seeking treatment when needed. When a woman has ambivalent symptoms The medical community may be slow to suspect ovarian cancer. This is especially true if the woman is at average risk or has no clear family history of the condition. Missed the opportunity to receive treatment early. and delayed diagnosis Part of the reason for this is ignorance.

deep ovarian position Lack of reliable screening Subtle and non-specific symptoms and misattributing symptoms to less severe conditions. All contribute to the delayed diagnosis of ovarian cancer. Treatment is less effective because of early intervention. More challenging Because ovarian cancer often doesn't show obvious symptoms until it has spread to other parts of the body, early detection is important. and ultimately improving survival rates. There is a need to increase awareness of the symptoms. Increase the ability to diagnose and promote early medical consultation.

How Ovarian Cancer Symptoms Overlap with Common Condition

Symptoms of ovarian cancer can mimic those of other diseases. More common This makes it a complex and often hidden disease. This is because symptoms are often vague and subtle. Therefore, early diagnosis So it's difficult. From a medical perspective It is important for patients and doctors to be aware of the similarities between the symptoms of ovarian cancer and those of benign gastrointestinal or gynecological disorders...

It's true that most ovarian cancer symptoms are similar to other symptoms. and less severe symptoms are one of the main obstacles to timely diagnosis. Bloating, abdominal pain, and changes in appetite or urination are some of the symptoms that patients may report. These symptoms are often seen in gastrointestinal disorders or other benign conditions, such as irritable bowel syndrome. For example, changes in urinary frequency can be misdiagnosed as a sign of an overactive bladder or a urinary tract infection. Urinate While bloating or feeling full can initially lead to digestive problems...

In addition, abnormal symptoms such as back pain, fatigue, and unexplained weight loss. which is a common symptom of other diseases It can be caused by ovarian cancer. If the patient has a history of other chronic diseases that cause similar symptoms, these systemic symptoms will not occur Suspected ovarian cancer immediately Especially when the cancer is still in its early stages and more treatable... Ovarian cancer can be difficult to distinguish at the pathophysiological level. This is because cancer is growing and spreading. As time passes Tumors can spread to nearby structures such as the intestines and peritoneum. Although it first appeared that there was a localized growth within the scrotum as the tumor grew, and causes the accumulation of ascites or fluid in the abdominal cavity. This can cause abdominal discomfort and swelling.

The gradual and progressive nature of ovarian cancer is an important feature that can help distinguish it from other diseases. Ovarian cancer often manifests as symptoms that worsen and worsen over time. This is different from digestive problems or hormonal fluctuations. This may have a cyclical or irregular pattern. This slow evolution may increase suspicion of malignancy. This is especially true when combined with other clinical findings, such as abnormal imaging or pelvic exams, connected to The importance of a comprehensive and nuanced clinical assessment is emphasized by covering the symptoms of ovarian cancer and ultimately the more prevalent condition. When symptoms do not go away or improve with standard treatment Medical professionals will need a broader range of differential diagnosis. It also depends on accurate detection. This can only be done by understanding the specific ways in which symptoms appear and change…

Recognizing Persistent Symptoms: The Key to Early Diagnosis and Survival

An important component of clinical practice is the recognition of ongoing symptoms. This is especially true in the case of complex diseases such as ovarian cancer. Ovarian cancer is referred to as "Silent killers" pose significant diagnostic challenges due to non-specific symptoms that often overlap with benign or less severe conditions. Despite these problems Early diagnosis, treatment, and ultimately good patient outcomes depend on the ability to Recognize consistent symptoms that are not temporary… and do not go away on their own.

Basically The importance of identifying persistent symptoms comes from their ability to serve as an early indicator of pathology that requires clinical examination. This is especially important in the case of ovarian cancer. In the early stages of ovarian cancer They often have no symptoms or have vague and unclear symptoms. Symptoms such as bloating, abdominal pain, and urinary urgency are common in women. It is often mistaken for benign conditions such as premenstrual syndrome (PMS) or irritable bowel syndrome (IBS), as symptoms often disappear with age. normal body fluctuations or mild gastrointestinal problems Incorrect positioning leads to delayed diagnosis. But an important clinical indicator that should spur further research is the long-term persistence of symptoms.

This is due to the lack of specific symptoms early on. and there is no effective screening tool for the general public. Ovarian cancer often presents at an advanced stage. This makes continued symptom awareness clinically important. different from breast cancer There is currently no widely accepted screening method for ovarian cancer.In stages III and IV, when the prognosis is not very good and the tumor has already spread. Preventing these delayed diagnoses requires the ability to recognize when symptoms persist longer or when they are more severe than is normal for a particular condition....

For example, chronic bloating is accompanied by other symptoms such as lower abdominal pain or frequent urination. This is often written up as a sign of malnutrition or gastrointestinal distress. It could be a sign of ovarian cancer. These symptoms may indicate a developing disease process that requires a more complete evaluation if they continue for weeks or months without interruption. This is now necessary because it can result in imaging tests such as an MRI, CT scan or pelvic ultrasound, as well as blood tests such as the CA-125 test when paired with the appropriate medical assessment These diagnostic tools can help identify early-stage ovarian cancer. Even though I didn't come to my own conclusions...

From a pathophysiological point of view Chronic symptoms often indicate the establishment or spread of the disease process. In the case of ovarian cancer, the tumor grows without any obvious symptoms at first. But when you grow up It begins to press on nearby structures such as the bladder or rectum. This can cause bowel or urinary changes. Abnormal condition that self-corrects both at the local and systematic levels Various processes Related to the biology of ovarian cancer And the continued appearance of resistance to treatment may indicate that the disease has progressed to the point where therapeutic intervention is required...

Moreover, It is impossible to overstate the behavioral and psychological components in determining persistent symptoms. Patients often show a pattern of treatment discontinuation or delay. This is especially true when symptoms are unclear or there is no clear cause. They may be reluctant to seek additional medical help. They blame stress or lifestyle choices for their discomfort. In these situations It is important to inform patients and medical professionals of the importance of persistence of symptoms. This is a sign that further diagnostic testing is required. early intervention It is important to improve clinical outcomes. and reduce the mental suffering of patients Not detecting a serious condition such as ovarian cancer can cause anxiety and hopelessness. It can build patients' confidence and improve their quality of life.

Treatment of ovarian cancer is also significantly influenced by the recognition of ongoing symptoms. The main treatment for ovarian cancer is surgery. This is often followed by chemotherapy. Adjuvant chemotherapy can further reduce the risk of recurrence. And the success rate of surgery for early-stage ovarian cancer (stages I and II) is relatively high. Early detection of ovarian cancer significantly improves survival outcomes. The five-year survival rate for stage I ovarian cancer is close to 90%, while the survival rate for stage III and IV ovarian cancer drops sharply. Therefore, a patient's prognosis and survival can change dramatically with ongoing symptoms. As a result, there are options for early detection and treatment.

in clinical practice A high index of suspicion is required for early detection of persistent symptoms. This is especially true in patients who are more likely to develop ovarian cancer, such as those with genetic mutations (such as BRCA1/2) or a family history of breast cancer. or ovarian cancer changes) even though the symptoms are clear But doctors must watch out for ovarian cancer in these situations. This is especially true for medical professionals who may be treating patients with unclear urinary or gastrointestinal symptoms. Inadequate detection of these symptoms can lead to delayed diagnosis and poorer outcomes. Therefore, when symptoms do not resolve within the clinically anticipated time, Doctors need to be trained to recognize patterns of symptoms beyond symptoms. and prioritize the diagnosis.

In the end Being able to recognize the lingering symptoms of ovarian cancer is important. This is because they can have a huge influence on early detection and treatment. This ultimately improves patient outcomes. Although symptoms of ovarian cancer are often vague and mild, But it should not be overlooked because symptoms persist. Healthcare professionals need to be aware that these symptoms may indicate the presence of cancer. This must be screened quickly and carefully. Early detection And appropriate surgery and chemotherapy can greatly improve a patient's survival rate and quality of life. To improve early diagnosis of disease and reduce the death rate from ovarian cancer It is important to raise awareness of the importance of persistent symptoms in patients and healthcare professionals.

Part 3

Advocating for early detection

Clinically, early detection of ovarian cancer is encouraged. It is a strategic approach to improving patient outcomes. Instead of promoting early diagnosis This is because ovarian cancer is often especially dangerous in its later stages. When cancer has spread outside the ovary, less than 30% are at stage 4, indicating a significantly reduced chance of survival due to later detection. Therefore, early detection therefore it is important But because there is no standard screening test and the symptoms are not clear. Therefore causing difficult problems as well.

According to medical experts The challenge with ovarian cancer lies in its appearance. Many non-serious symptoms include irritable bowel syndrome (IBS), menstrual changes. A urinary tract infection (UTI) can cause symptoms such as bloating, abdominal pain, and changes in bowel or urination habits. Patients often ignore these symptoms. And medical professionals may not notice. Especially if the symptoms are mild or sporadic... or so Ovarian cancer often does not have symptoms that indicate other types of cancer, such as a noticeable lump. or clear diagnostic indications. As a result, it is challenging to distinguish benign causes of these symptoms from potentially dangerous causes.

From the perspective of medical professionals There needs to be a balance between promoting early detection. and increasing awareness and avoiding overdiagnosis. Doctors need to be aware of the risk of ovarian cancer. This is especially true in patients at high risk, such as with known genetic mutations such as BRCA1 or BRCA2, or with a family history of the disease However, for the general public Doctors must exercise caution in recommending unnecessary tests. If there is no clear information This is because there is no breast cancer screening method that works for everyone like a standard mammogram. Clinicians are therefore wary of relying solely on imaging studies such as ultrasound or blood tests such as CA-125, which can result in false positives and unnecessary procedures...

In practice Doctors must balance the need for early detection. Given the reality of resource constraints, for example, identifying persisting symptoms and beginning the diagnostic process is extremely valuable. But the healthcare system is often overburdened. And doctors must consider more than just clinical data in making decisions. as well as prioritizing disease screening with preventive measures, access to resources and clear policies. In this context, there is a need to increase the awareness of the public and medical community about this disease. To remove barriers to preventing early diagnosis of ovarian cancer...

Building trust among patients and health care providers is also essential for doctors' support in early detection. If the ongoing symptoms are not immediately related to something more serious like cancer. Women may not always be aware of the significance of such symptoms. To reassure patients that taking care of their own health is acceptable. and early diagnosis of disease considered important Even if it's something less serious. Doctors should speak clearly and empathetically. Patients are more likely to be involved in the diagnostic process when they feel heard and understood. This results in faster intervention and better outcomes...

To sum up, from a medical standpoint, promoting early ovarian cancer detection is crucial to raising survival rates and lowering the disease's overall burden. Physicians must manage risk Factors: Educate patients and refer patients for appropriate diagnosis. In addition to identifying consistent symptoms Early detection of ovarian cancer can change it significantly. From life-threatening diagnoses to treatable and manageable diseases. This support for medical professionals goes beyond a simple diagnosis. Its aim is to empower women to take control of their health. This ultimately results in better and more efficient care.

Although such strategies are part of a larger public health framework, which covers cancer prevention Early diagnosis Choosing treatment and healthcare infrastructure The World Health Organization (WHO) plays an important role in promoting early detection of ovarian cancer. and improve outcomes for women around the world. The organization recognizes that ovarian cancer is a major barrier to early detection. This is especially true in low-resource environments. Because most symptoms are subtle and vague, the WHO strategy for ovarian cancer does not only focus on direct diagnostic steps. but also focuses on strengthening the international health system.

Promoting education and awareness about cancer is a key component of WHO's involvement. This is important because symptoms of ovarian cancer can be misdiagnosed because many women are unaware or overlook it as a problem. Not dangerous Increase your knowledge of possible symptoms of ovarian cancer. Including changes in bowel or urinary behavior. Chronic bloating and abdominal pain. Try to learn. With this study, people, especially women in high-risk groups Have the power to get treatment as quickly as possible. Instead of waiting until symptoms worsen or you become incapacitated To increase rates of early intervention, WHO is also working to raise awareness to ensure that medical professionals know and can see these subtle warning indicators.

WHO also emphasizes the importance of strengthening health systems, especially in low- and middle-income countries where access to health services may be limited. The health care system must have the necessary infrastructure. Qualified medical staff and adequate diagnostic tools for early intervention to detect ovarian cancer. Fast and efficient Advanced diagnostic tools, such as imaging technology or blood tests (such as CA-125), are not available in many countries. This is especially true for resource-limited countries, and WHO encourages the introduction of inexpensive and easily accessible diagnostic techniques into the healthcare system to close this gap. This strategy ensures early diagnosis. Regardless of a woman's economic status, WHO also supports raising the standard of healthcare infrastructure to enable accurate diagnosis and appropriate referral. It ensures that ovarian cancer is not neglected in areas with limited access to specialized treatment.

WHO's support for cancer prevention and risk reduction is a key component of this strategy. Although there are no universal screening guidelines for ovarian cancer, WHO supports a more comprehensive approach to reducing the overall burden of cancer. This includes educating women about known risk factors. and promote awareness of reproductive health related to ovarian cancer. For example, the World Health Organization supports programs that inform women of the benefits of using contraception. This has been shown to reduce the risk of ovarian cancer. WHO also promotes genetic testing and counseling for women who are genetically likely to be at high risk, such as those with families. History of breast or ovarian cancer Identification of women at genetic risk allows for preventative measures. Early detection and more targeted surveillance.

Finally, the World Health Organization emphasizes the importance of ensuring access to palliative care and treatment. Many women find it difficult to access high quality treatment. This is especially true in areas with limited resources. Even in high-income countries where ovarian cancer may be detected earlier, WHO Cancer Care ensures that women with ovarian cancer have access to needed treatment, such as surgery and chemotherapy, regardless of location or medical status. economy As well as promoting a more equitable approach, WHO recognizes that patients with serious illnesses need better supportive care to reduce symptoms and improve their quality of life.

In summary, WHO's support for early detection of ovarian cancer is supported. It is part of a larger public health framework that aims to raise awareness. improve access to treatment Strengthen the health care system and reduce the risk of cancer WTO Efforts to Prevent Cancer Strengthening the health system and giving knowledge is extremely important To improve outcomes for women around the world, WHO hopes to create a global environment in which ovarian cancer is detected early. Treated more successfully and improve access to care and support focused on these comprehensive initiatives..

The importance of self-awareness
Especially when it comes to diseases like ovarian cancer, self-awareness regular health check And being able to report when things aren't going your way is an important component of personal health management. Empowering people to take care of their health These practices not only help with early diagnosis but also have the potential to improve outcomes and prevent serious illness from developing…

The first step in understanding your body and identifying potential problems is developing self-awareness. Many diseases, including early-stage ovarian cancer, Have mild or vague symptoms If you know the specific state of your body You'll be able to better identify when something goes off or continues. Over time, for example, observing general or expected changes in bowel and urinary tract behavior, bloating, abdominal pain, or past symptoms. It may indicate that further research is needed. Self-awareness also involves being aware of changes in your overall health. Be it emotional or physical. These changes are normal. Aspects of aging or stress... It goes without saying that there are many different conditions, including ovarian cancer. Early detection Depend on your body's signals and trust your instincts.

Another important component of maintaining good health and preventing disease is regular checkups. Appointments with your health care provider are an important time for professional evaluation. Mentoring and teaching are not the only standard performance possibilities. Doctors can perform diagnostic tests, physical examinations, and provide medical knowledge that others cannot receive. Although there is no universal screening for women with ovarian cancer who are asymptomatic, If you still have symptoms or have risk factors Doctors can also perform a comprehensive assessment. Patients can also ask questions during routine checkups. Discuss concerns and ask for advice about lifestyle choices Risk factor management and preventive health measures...

One of the most important first steps in promoting your own health is reporting when something is wrong. When their symptoms seem vague or unimportant Many people tend to discount these symptoms or are unwilling to discuss them with a doctor. But communicating concerns, no matter how small, is important for identifying more serious health problems early. Talking with a health care professional about discomfort, unusual symptoms, or changes in body processes can lead to further research and possibly early diagnosis. This is because early symptoms of ovarian cancer can be mistaken for more common and less severe symptoms. It is therefore important to remember that there are no symptoms at all. Too small to mention like a feeling; It is also an important step to ensure that your health is properly assessed and treated.

These behaviors include talking and regular check-ups. and self-awareness They are valuable because they can shift the paradigm of the health care system from being reactive to being more proactive. You can take care of your health and play your part in the prevention and detection of diseases like ovarian cancer. Be aware of changes in your body and consult your doctor if anything unusual occurs. The chances of a problem being treatable and having a positive outcome increase when the problem is identified early. Learning and understanding these behaviors can promote a strong culture. Where people feel comfortable talking about their health and wellbeing. A proactive approach to health is important to improving general quality of life. as well as preventing serious illness for everyone. especially women They must understand the importance of expressing their opinions on health issues. and how regular communication with health professionals can impact long-term health trajectories.

Talk to your doctor if you find out any symptoms

Open, honest, and constructive communication is important when discussing symptoms with your doctor. This is especially true if you're worried about things like ovarian cancer or suspect something is wrong. It's important to remember that no symptom is too minor to talk about and there are doctors available to help. By providing the doctor with an accurate and realistic description of your symptoms. The doctor can then give you the best treatment.

First of all, prepare yourself for your visit. Write down symptoms, duration, and other relevant information such as when they occurred. severity of symptoms and whether it interferes with your daily activities or not. This plan guarantees that you will not forget any important information. And it helps you stay organized throughout the conversation. For example, if you've lost weight for no apparent reason, Excretion behavior has changed. or chronic bloating Describe how long these symptoms lasted. and whether the symptoms worsen over time If you can be more specific and detailed about what you are experiencing. Your doctor can Evaluate the situation more accurately…able

It is also important to communicate your concerns in a simple and understandable way. Let your doctor know that you are concerned about the possible causes of these symptoms. Especially if it's unfamiliar or different from previous experiences. You can say something like "No matter what I eat or how much I exercise, I've been bloated for several weeks now. and it doesn't seem to go away." It's unusual for me, so I'm worried. Don't be afraid to express your concerns about ovarian cancer or other special symptoms. In addition to helping to resolve symptoms, your doctor can better address your concerns if they are aware of your thoughts.

It's important to ask open-ended questions so you can fully understand your health status during the conversation. You can ask questions like or "What tests or procedures do you recommend to help identify the problem?" rather than "Is this serious?" This approach helps you understand the medical reasons for your doctor's recommendation. In addition to providing access to more complete answers. Don't be afraid to ask how the diagnostic tests recommended by your doctor can help you determine the source of your symptoms. To understand your treatment options, read "How do these tests work?" and "If the results show a specific situation What must I do next?"

It is also important to ask about the next steps of the process. Especially if you are unsure of the diagnosis. If the doctor recommends a course of action Ask about the expected follow-up time or the duration of results. For example, when receiving a possible diagnosis, you would ask, "What should I do while I wait for the test results?" or "What if nothing else?" serious What are the treatment options?" These questions ensure you are not left with unanswered questions and help you understand the seriousness of the situation.

It is very important to bring any past medical history or risk factors that may be related to your current symptoms. It's a good idea to ask your doctor about the possible influence of existing medical conditions. genetic defect or family history It is important to ask about family history of ovarian or other cancers. This is because it may affect the type of test your doctor recommends. If you think your family history puts you at greater risk for a certain condition. Don't be afraid to ask about the role of genetic counseling.

Finally, be sure to ask about resources that can update and support you throughout the diagnosis process. Your therapist may recommend educational resources. support group or other medical professionals that specializes in your specific problem It's always helpful to get more information. This is especially true when dealing with complex medical issues. And having these resources at your disposal can help you make better decisions about your health...

In summary, getting the best care requires you to be proactive and open with your doctor about your symptoms and concerns. Observing symptoms Communicating Concerns And asking informed questions will help you prepare for your visit. This guarantees that your doctor has all the information needed to diagnose you. and your patients understand the process The rationale behind medical advice and the next step Openness, trust, and a thorough understanding of your health are the foundations of a successful conversation that will ultimately result. Better care and peace of mind

Detecting ovarian cancer early important note for woman

This is because the symptoms of ovarian cancer may not be obvious. and symptoms of other conditions May be easily misunderstood Identifying disease at an early stage is often challenging. But women can focus on some tips and behaviors that can help catch ovarian cancer early....

Chronic bloating is one of the first things a woman must consider. Bloating is normal for many women, but if it continues for a long time or occurs frequently it could be a sign of an ovarian problem. In addition to bloating, other symptoms This may include changes in appetite or feeling suddenly full after eating a small amount of food. Tumors that press on the stomach cause changes in appetite. And women feel full even after eating a small amount of food.

Persistent or persistent pelvic and abdominal pain can be an early warning sign. This type of pain can be blurry, such as a dull ache or pain in the lower abdomen. Women should be aware of bladder-related symptoms that can occur as a result of ovarian pressure, such as increased frequency or urgency to urinate...
Unexpected weight changes, such as sudden weight loss or gain. Should also be checked. This is because it may be caused by fluid retention associated with ovarian cancer. If a woman has irregular periods or menopausal bleeding. which is an example of the changes in her menstrual cycle...

Fatigue is severe exhaustion or lack of energy inconsistent with rest. This is another prominent symptom. This can occur as a result of metabolic changes or as the body fights disease. Additionally, because of ovarian cancer, gastrointestinal symptoms such as nausea, constipation, or bloating can sometimes be accompanied by gastrointestinal symptoms. Women should be careful of these symptoms as well...

Chronic back pain of unknown origin that is not related to any medical condition or exercise. It could be a sign of ovarian cancer. Talking with your doctor about genetic testing to check for inherited risk can be helpful for women at high risk, such as those with a family history of the disease. Breast or ovarian cancer

Finally, your doctor may perform a pelvic exam as part of your routine checkup to detect early ovarian abnormalities. Ovarian cancer may be detected with tests such as a vaginal ultrasound. and the CA-125 blood test, which measures specific blood proteins. Especially if symptoms persist or cause concern...

It's important to remember that while these symptoms are common in many different conditions, they can also be linked to ovarian cancer. Women should talk with a health care professional for an accurate diagnosis and evaluation. Instead of making a hasty decision

Part 4

Why ovarian cancer need more attention

This is because the symptoms are mild and there is a lack of early detection techniques. efficient Ovarian cancer is therefore still classified as a malignant gynecological cancer. and needs more care and attention Ovarian cancer often shows no outward symptoms at an early stage. which is different from some types of cancer When they do occur, these symptoms are often vague and may be mistaken for less serious illnesses such as bloating, abdominal pain, or loss of appetite. As a result, many women are diagnosed after their cancer has spread to other parts of the body, causing severe symptoms to decrease. Treatment options and survival rates...

Ovarian cancer is more difficult for the general public due to a lack of reliable screening tests. Although there are tests for the CA-125 marker, such as blood tests and intravaginal ultrasound, But they are not always reliable or effective at detecting early cancer. Most women are not diagnosed until their cancer has spread. At which point it becomes *more difficult to maintain.

Additionally, ovarian cancer research has historically received less funding than other types of cancer. This limits the development of early detection methods. and available treatments As a result, ovarian cancer survival rates have improved only slightly in the past decade. Understanding ovarian cancer and determining targeted treatments has become more complicated due to the complexity of the disease. This includes many subtypes and genetic makeup...

Ovarian cancer also disproportionately affects women. And the serious impact on families and communities is often overlooked. This silent killer needs more funding, research and awareness. And the emotional symptoms of this disease are often aggravated by challenging treatments. Greater investment in ovarian cancer research can increase early detection. Create more effective treatments And ultimately save more people's lives...

This is due to the difficulty in detection, treatment and overall prognosis. Ovarian cancer therefore urgently needs more attention from a treatment perspective. Micro-onset of ovarian cancer is one of the features that worries doctors, bloating, pelvic pain. And changes in bowel habits are examples of non-specific symptoms that are often mistaken for benign illnesses, such as premenstrual syndrome. or abnormalities of the digestive system Additionally, there is no effective screening test for ovarian cancer in the general population. This is despite great progress in cancer research. Ultrasound and serum markers such as CA-125 can help in the diagnosis. But it is not precise enough to identify the earliest and most treatable stages of the disease. Lack of prevalence and efficiency... Due to the testing process, many women are only diagnosed after the cancer has spread outside their ovaries. At the same time, there are few treatment options and a much worse prognosis...

Ovarian cancer is clinically complex due to its heterogeneity. Most cases are diagnosed as epithelial ovarian cancer. which are notoriously resistant to treatment Especially when detected at an advanced stage. But the disease can present itself in several subtypes. Each species has a unique biological behavior. The cornerstone of management remains maintaining standards. This includes surgery to remove the tissue and chemotherapy. However, survival rates have not improved significantly in recent decades. and the recurrence rate remains high. This emphasizes the need for more focused treatment. Individual treatment strategies and increase knowledge about the molecular causes of ovarian cancer...

Research into ovarian cancer does not receive as much funding or attention as other types of cancer. This hampers efforts to develop new treatments. and techniques for detecting cancer in its early stages As a medical expert We know that increasing funding, research, and awareness can result in discoveries and improvements. Possibility of detection This ultimately results in an increased survival rate. It is impossible to overestimate the emotional and psychological damage that ovarian cancer does to patients and their families. So improving outcomes doesn't just save lives. But it also helps reduce emotional problems. From all these considerations It is therefore essential to increase awareness about ovarian cancer. Providing education and funding to increase early detection available treatments And finally, the patient's results...

Lack of public awareness on ovarian cancer

Several studies around the world have shown that women are more likely to be diagnosed with advanced ovarian cancer. When treatment is challenging and public awareness of the disease is low The main reason for late presentation or delayed diagnosis has been cited as a lack of public awareness of early stage ovarian cancer, cancer symptoms, and cancer symptoms.

One major barrier to early detection and treatment of ovarian cancer is the general lack of knowledge about the disease. Early symptoms of ovarian cancer are mild and may be easily missed or mistaken for benign disease. This is one of the main causes of lack of awareness. Nausea, abdominal pain, and frequent urination A common symptom of many other benign diseases, they stop treatment. The general public's limited understanding of ovarian cancer is also the result of a lack of open discussion in the media and public health initiatives.. .

Many women learn about ovarian cancer too late. Usually after symptoms get so bad that the cancer has spread outside the ovaries. This makes treatment more difficult and less successful. This postponement of medical treatment is largely due to women's ignorance. Risk factors include age, BRCA genetic mutations and family history. If women are not aware of these risks or early warning signs, They may not understand how important it is to see a doctor when they have symptoms...

Another factor contributing to this problem is the lack of reliable and widespread screening for ovarian cancer. Methods for early detection of ovarian cancer are not universally effective. It's like breast or cervical cancer. which has screening techniques such as mammograms or Pap smears In the absence of a proactive screening program Women must rely on their ability to recognize symptoms. As noted above, this can be vague and confusing. Inadequate public awareness of this topic often leads to risky delays in diagnosis. Which directly affects the survival rate...

The stigma associated with gynecological cancer compounds compounds the lack of knowledge by discouraging some women from speaking openly about their symptoms or seeking help. Many women avoid needed medical advice because they feel embarrassed or uncomfortable talking about issues such as pelvic pain or changes in digestive health. Later diagnosis results From a combination of subtle symptoms Lack of public awareness and there is a lack of broad study on this matter. increasing education Raise public awareness and implement proactive health programs that emphasize the value of early detection. and the need for women to Focus on their body

How you can help family and friends [love ones]

Educating your friends and loved ones about ovarian cancer is important to promote early detection. and save people's lives Open communication and education are two powerful ways to help. Promoting conversations about family medical history can help others identify subtle markers that might otherwise go unnoticed by providing reliable, well-researched information about ovarian cancer factors. Risks, symptoms, and the importance of early detection And encouraging regular health check-ups can also help. Loved ones need to take care of their own health.

A great way to raise awareness is through social media. You can reach a larger audience and start a conversation about the importance of recognizing the early signs of ovarian cancer by sharing educational posts, articles, videos, or even personal stories about the disease. Infographics and other visual campaigns Facts or symptoms about ovarian cancer that catch people's attention are easy to share. You can also join or start an ovarian cancer awareness group. where participants can exchange resources Stories from direct experience and emotional support Using hashtags like #ListenToYourBody or #OvarianCancerAwareness It can help coordinate your efforts and ensure that more people see the message.

Supporting organizations and initiatives related to ovarian cancer can also make a significant impact. You can support research Advanced rapid detection techniques And ultimately save lives by donating. Participate in awareness raising activities such as walking or running. Or taking your time...

Providing emotional support to those affected by ovarian cancer is also important. A compassionate listen, going to the doctor, or even helping with daily tasks can be very helpful if you know someone who is sick. Their emotional burden can be reduced. And they have confidence in taking care of their health with your help....

We can help educate others. Reduce the stigma associated with gynecological cancer. and promote early detection and ultimately better outcomes for women with ovarian cancer using connected personal and public platforms.

In addition to improving early detection, increasing public knowledge about ovarian cancer is also important in educating the public about the condition. Destroy false beliefs and promote preventive health practices. Our loved ones and communities will be better prepared to face ovarian cancer if we have more of them. Conversation about it and its difficulties

Sharing first-hand stories or anecdotes of people affected by ovarian cancer is a powerful way to raise awareness. Showing others what it's like to live with or support someone with ovarian cancer. These stories can humanize the disease. Posting these stories on social media can attract readers and encourage them to seek treatment if they experience similar symptoms. These stories can serve as a reminder to those affected that they are not alone and promote a sense of community.

Sharing educational resources has become easier with social media platforms. Several organizations, including the National Ovarian Cancer Coalition and Ovarian Cancer Research Alliance, are dedicated to raising awareness of ovarian cancer and network of organizations share articles, blog posts, videos, and interviews with experts. They provide reliable and helpful resources about symptoms, risk factors, and are available. Family history Genetic testing (such as BRCA) for chronic inflammation pelvic pain Difficulty eating and the importance of recognizing symptoms such as urinary urgency. Here are some examples of how these resources can play an important role in teaching. How to recognize early warning signs and encourage regular doctor visits.

Another effective strategy for getting your community involved is to host awareness events in person or online. This could be anything from planning a small fundraiser or walking to raise awareness in your community. to hosting a live stream on social media with an ovarian cancer expert. In addition to creating awareness These gatherings also provide an opportunity for people to express their concerns, ask questions and receive information about ovarian cancer prevention...

Research, early detection techniques And creating better treatment options can be directly impacted by funding ovarian cancer organizations through donations or fundraising events. You can encourage others to donate or get involved by spreading the word in your community about the importance of other initiatives.

Another valuable way to help is to offer support to friends and loved ones affected by ovarian cancer. It is important to provide an emotional and physical support network to those you care about who have been diagnosed with the disease. Providing a compassionate listening ear or helping with a doctor's appointment can sometimes reduce stress. Knowing they have a loved one who struggles with fear or loneliness can make a huge difference to an ovarian cancer patient. You can also help them with daily tasks or research treatment options to help them focus on their health.

Combating the stigma associated with gynecological cancer is another important component of raising awareness. Talking about issues related to the reproductive system can be uncomfortable or embarrassing for many women. By promoting open discussion about ovarian cancer and showing others that it is acceptable to discuss these issues. We can encourage women to talk about their health and seek medical advice when needed. This is especially important because women may feel embarrassed talking about their ovarian cancer symptoms. This is because their symptoms are often mistaken for other illnesses. Less serious...

Finally, try integrating awareness raising activities into regular conversations. Bringing up the topic of ovarian cancer in casual conversation or encouraging friends and family to adopt preventive health practices. It can help normalize conversations about gynecological health. Ask about family medical history Support regular health examinations and keep an eye on changes in their health In the end Your proactive approach can save lives by promoting a culture of self-care and early detection.

You can help remove barriers to early diagnosis and treatment. Research support and promote a supportive environment for those affected by ovarian cancer by combining these efforts: Education share resources Provide support to those affected and disease by talking frankly and openly Regarding the topic, by doing this you will reduce the stigma. Create important awareness and ensuring that ovarian cancer receives much-needed care and funding.

Part 5

Understanding your body

An important component of maintaining overall health is being aware of your body. This is especially true when looking for possible signs of ovarian cancer or other diseases. Promoting self-awareness and enabling women to recognize changes that may indicate a problem are key elements in helping. They are more in tune with their bodies. In the fight against ovarian cancer This is often discovered in advanced stages because the symptoms are minor and easily missed. Such awareness allows for early detection. which is important...

Understanding what stands out to you is the first step to becoming more aware of your body. Because every woman's body is different. Knowing your normal characteristics such as your menstrual cycle, eating habits, and energy levels It will help recognize deviations that may indicate a problem. This includes constantly monitoring your body's sensations. Noticing new symptoms or strange symptoms all the time... also including understanding that it doesn't feel right...

For example, it is important to recognize symptoms such as chronic bloating. pelvic pain Unexplained changes in appetite, frequent urination, or abdominal pain, although ovarian cancer is often associated with these symptoms. But it can also be a symptom of other illnesses. It is important if symptoms persist or get worse over time. This should be discussed with a health professional. This is because symptoms of early stage ovarian cancer often mimic those of less serious conditions, such as menstrual cramps or indigestion. The disease is therefore difficult to diagnose when the symptoms deviate from the typical experience. And women who are familiar with their normal body rhythms are better equipped to recognize and seek treatment. Quickly...

Learning your family medical history is another important part of understanding your body. The risk of ovarian cancer may increase with genetic predisposition, such as mutations in the BRCA1 or BRCA2 genes. Breast and ovarian cancers are more common in women with a family history of the disease. If you are aware of your genetic risks You can discuss routine screening or genetic testing with your healthcare provider.

Living a healthy lifestyle, which can reduce your risk of ovarian cancer, is another aspect of treating your body. You can keep your body healthy by eating a balanced diet. Exercise often Manage stress And avoid smoking and drinking too much alcohol. In addition to making women more aware of their own bodies, This holistic approach to health also reduces the chance of contracting serious diseases.

Women who engage in self-care techniques such as yoga, meditation, and mindfulness You can also develop a stronger bond with your body. By teaching people to be more aware of their own experiences. These techniques help them identify physical discomfort or changes in body sensation. This may indicate a hidden problem...

In the end The key to understanding your body is open communication with your healthcare provider. Women who are proactive about their health will benefit from regular checkups. This includes a pelvic exam and counseling regarding any symptoms or changes. It is important to discuss any concerns or unusual symptoms with your doctor during these visits. Women will feel more comfortable with their health. and feel more confident to seek advice or treatment when needed. If they have a trusted relationship with a health care provider

We help women take control of their health and identify potential problems early. By teaching them to be more aware of their own bodies. Understanding your body involves more than just your response to symptoms. It also includes preventative measures such as tracking changes. Seeking medical help when needed and creating healthy routines that support long-term health. Ultimately, this strategy can lead to better health outcomes. and increases survival rates for ovarian cancer and other diseases

Regular exercise is essential for early detection of health problems. including ovarian cancer and is an important foundation of proactive health management. A woman can assess her general well-being. Track changes in your health over time. and deal with potential risks before they become serious. first line of defense When more can be treated and early intervention It is important to improve results...

One of the main benefits of regular checkups is that they allow medical professionals to keep an eye on and assess your health even when you are feeling better. Many diseases, such as cancers such as ovarian cancer, often develop silently. and there is no external signal Regular visits to your health care provider can be examined, tested, and tested, which can help identify potential health problems you may not be aware of, such as: Regular pelvic exams. Talking with your doctor about family history and risk factors can help identify warnings about ovarian cancer. Signals from the beginning Even though all women There is no universal test method for all woman

A comprehensive evaluation of reproductive health, including pelvic and breast exams as well as conversations regarding menstrual health, should be part of women's checkups. Any abnormalities in the menstrual cycle or unusual symptoms such as bloating, abdominal pain, or urinary problems can be evaluated by a healthcare professional. These symptoms may be linked to ovarian cancer or other gynecological concerns. These routine examinations offer a chance to address issues that may appear minor or unrelated to cancer, but are crucial to a woman's overall health.

Regular screening provides an important screening test that can help identify additional health risks, such as diabetes, high blood pressure, or heart disease, in addition to reproductive health. When women get older These tests are especially important because chronic conditions can be detected earlier and can be managed better. To reduce the risk of cancer and other diseases. Your doctor can also give you advice on how to manage stress. How to maintain a healthy weight and decide on other healthy lifestyle choices...

Additionally, routine screening provides a forum to discuss genetic testing. Family history and personal risk factors. For example, women with a family history of breast or ovarian cancer should talk with their doctor about genetic testing options, such as BRCA testing. These discussions are important to understanding health risks. of the individual and develop strategies for early detection or prevention. Your doctor may recommend more frequent screenings or preventive measures. In the case of a genetic predisposition To reduce the risk of ovarian cancer...

Another important component of regular checkups is mental health. Many women are conscious about their health. But they may be reluctant to talk about it in appointments. Regular doctor's appointments provide an opportunity to discuss emotional health. Reduce worry about potential medical problems and asking for advice on managing mental health A more comprehensive approach to health is guaranteed when mental and physical health are addressed together.

In addition to physical examination and screening Women may also be asked questions about their health during the exam. These conversations can encourage women to take charge of their health. and help identify physical changes that may need attention. Screening increases the chance of detecting potential problems early. It provides an opportunity to correct any unusual symptoms or concerns. As soon as it appears

It all comes down to regular checkups to understand your body. Identify potential health problems and receive timely treatment These counseling sessions are important for maintaining long-term health. whether it is chronic disease management or early detection of silent diseases such as ovarian cancer, women can be confident that they are informed about their health. And take the necessary precautions to avoid developing a serious condition undetected by prioritizing regular screening....

It's important to Know your family history

This is because genetic factors can be passed on from generation to generation. Family history therefore is important in developing ovarian cancer. In relation to ovarian cancer Family history means the likelihood of the disease affecting family members. Especially those closely related, such as a mother's sister or daughter, are associated with the possibility of inherited genetic mutations that increase the risk of ovarian cancer.

Mutations in the BRCA1 and BRCA2 genes are well-known genetic factors. Normally, these genes help repair damaged DNA, but when they mutate, These genes cause uncontrolled cell growth. This may result in cancer. A woman's risk of ovarian cancer is significantly higher. This is often much higher than in the general population. If she inherits mutations in these genes genes from one of her parents, such as BRCA1. The lifetime risk of ovarian cancer for women with the mutation is between 40% and 60%, which is higher than the average risk of 1-2% in the general population. In the same way BRCA2 mutations also increase your risk. Although generally to a lesser extent.
A person's risk increases if they have a family history of ovarian cancer. This is especially true if several close relatives have this disease. If ovarian cancer runs in the family The genetic mutation is likely to continue for generations. This may indicate a genetic predisposition to the condition. For example, a woman is more likely to develop ovarian cancer herself if her mother or sister has ovarian cancer. The risk increases further when multiple immediate relatives (mothers, sisters or daughters) are affected. This indicates a strong genetic link. In these situations The underlying cause may be a genetic mutation, such as that found in the BRCA gene.

Additionally, ethnicity may influence genetic risk factors for ovarian cancer, for example, compared to women from other ethnic groups. Ashkenazi Jewish women are known to have a higher prevalence of BRCA1 and BRCA2 mutations, and if these mutations run in their family, They may be at increased risk for ovarian cancer....

Many women with a strong family history of ovarian cancer may seek genetic counseling or undergo genetic testing because of a genetic link. These tests can determine if a BRCA1 or BRCA2 mutation is present. If a genetic mutation is discovered, It may provide important information to directly assist in decision-making about preventive measures, such as improving ovarian cancer surveillance, medication use, or significantly reducing the risk of ovarian cancer...

All things considered A family history of ovarian cancer is an important indicator that may be related to genetic factors. It can help inform choices about genetic testing and possible preventive measures. and increases the chance that the family may have inherited mutations that increase risk. If only people were aware of the link between ovarian cancer and family history. They are able to make better health decisions and have better control over their risks.

Talking with your health care provider about your family history and ovarian cancer is important in determining your personal risk and helping you make decisions about your health. You can determine that you are at increased risk for ovarian cancer due to genetic factors. Family history or other concerns Related or not By having an open and honest conversation with your health care provider...

It is important to provide as much specific information as possible to your health care provider about your family history of ovarian cancer. This includes informing family members who have ovarian cancer, especially your mother, sister, daughter and other immediate relatives, as well as the age at diagnosis. Your healthcare provider will be able to better determine whether you are at high risk for this disease.

Additional information If you have other types of cancer in your family, such as breast cancer or colon cancer. or endometrial cancer Your doctor may also want to know about these cancers. This is because many types of cancer have a genetic component. Having multiple types of cancer in a family can indicate an inherited trait, such as Lynch syndrome or a BRCA1 or BRCA2 mutation, which increases the risk of ovarian cancer. Knowing your family history of different types of cancer It is important because of these inherited characteristics. A person's cancer risk has a huge impact on their lifetime.

Your doctor can assess your genetic risk for ovarian cancer by asking about your family history. They may recommend genetic counseling and testing if they find that your family history puts you at greater risk. BRCA1, BRCA2, and other gene mutations associated with a higher risk of ovarian cancer are among those. Specific mutations sought by genetic testing Tests can better understand your risk. And if the mutation is discovered There may be options for surgery to reduce risk or, more often, monitoring.

It is also important to share information about your personal health and any symptoms you may be having. Detecting ovarian cancer in its early stages can be challenging. Because the symptoms are not clear This includes bloating, abdominal pain, and changes in bowel habits. If you have a family history of ovarian cancer and display these symptoms Your doctor may test or More frequent imaging to keep an eye on your ovarian health so they can be tested or advised

In addition to genetic testing Discussing your family history with your doctor can help you decide how to best manage your risks. Your doctor may consider options such as more frequent pelvic exams, ultrasounds, or preventative treatments. If you are found to be at high risk of ovarian cancer Preventative procedures such as oophorectomy can be considered in some cases. Especially if you are sure that your genetic risk is high.

Talking about your family history of ovarian cancer can help you identify your potential risks. You can take an active part in managing your health by discussing your family history with your health care provider. Discussion about lifestyle changes Early detection techniques and preventative care that can reduce the risk of ovarian cancer. or detected early When more can be treated This can be facilitated by the information you provide...

Finally, discussing your family history with your doctor is important in determining your risk. Look at potential preventative surveillance. and early detection strategies This fosters a collaborative relationship where you and your health care provider can jointly develop a customized health management plan based on your specific genetic risks and family history.

Part 6

Life after ovarian cancer:Coping with side effects

In the past few years Ovarian cancer diagnoses and deaths are decreasing. Meanwhile, the number of individuals living with and apart from the disease increases. Recovering from pre-ovarian cancer can be difficult. There are short-term and long-term side effects associated with treatment. Some of which may not be curable. The high recurrence of ovarian cancer can be a cause for concern.

Coping with short-term side effects

Chemotherapy and surgery are commonly used to treat ovarian cancer. If additional treatment is required It can be detected through genetic testing." If genetic testing shows a BRCA mutation, the patient may be eligible for maintenance medication called a PARP inhibitor in an attempt to maintain symptom relief. These drugs are given to patients approximately two years after chemotherapy."

Dealing with the short-term side effects of ovarian cancer treatment can be challenging. But understanding treatments and how to control visible symptoms is essential in trying to eradicate cancer and extend life. Treatment for ovarian cancer usually involves a combination of chemotherapy and surgery. They can have Serious negative consequences.

Surgery is often the first line of treatment for ovarian cancer. Surgery aims to remove as much of the tumor as possible. and usually involves the removal of the uterus, ovaries, and surrounding tissue. or other surrounding lymph nodes, depending on how far the cancer has spread Surgery usually involves chemotherapy after surgery to eradicate it completely. Cancer cells that still exist Chemotherapy works well to target cells that are dividing quickly. But it is not effective only against cancer cells. Additionally, the body may lose healthy cells, which can result in a number of specific side effects. Even if you get enough sleep Fatigue is normal and can be overwhelming. Chemotherapy can also result in nausea, vomiting, and loss of appetite. This makes it difficult to eat and stay energized. Another well-known side effect that can be difficult for patients both emotionally and physically is hair loss. Chemotherapy can also result in mouth sores that make eating and swallowing difficult. As well as suppressing the immune system makes patients more vulnerable to infection...

Self-care techniques and medical intervention are used to manage these side effects. Medicine can prevent nausea. And fatigue can be managed with dietary changes or increased hydration. Palliative care is provided by medical experts and teams. Including counseling, physical therapy and dietary advice. To help reduce the discomfort associated with treatment...

In addition to surgery and chemotherapy Genetic testing is also part of treatment for ovarian cancer. Testing for genetic mutations, such as in the BRCA1 and BRCA2 genes, can help determine whether patients will benefit from additional treatment after chemotherapy. with the detection of inherited mutations that increase the risk of ovarian cancer. These genetic tests help determine the most effective treatment plan. For example, if genetic testing reveals that a patient has a BRCA mutation, a PARP inhibitor may be prescribed as part of the patient's treatment.

A new class of drugs called PARP inhibitors is used as maintenance therapy after chemotherapy. These drugs work by blocking the PARP enzyme, which helps repair damaged DNA in cells. Interfering with DNA repair prevents cancer cells from surviving and spreading. Especially cells that have been damaged by chemotherapy. For patients with BRCA mutations, PARP inhibitors may be a necessary treatment to prolong cancer remission. These drugs are generally taken for two years after chemotherapy. and found to greatly increase survival rates

Despite great advances in the treatment of ovarian cancer, But PARP inhibitors come with their own set of potential side effects. Although many patients still experience these side effects, But these symptoms are generally not as severe as the side effects of chemotherapy. Patients may experience side effects such as fatigue and mild nausea. and changes in the number of red blood cells This may increase your risk of infection or anemia. Some patients may be more sensitive to blood clots while taking these medications. Despite these potential side effects, PARP inhibitors are a new treatment that has been shown to maintain symptomatic relief and improve long-term outcomes for women with ovarian cancer that has undergone mutations. Variants of BRCA

Managing the short-term side effects of treatment requires a comprehensive approach that considers both the mental and physical aspects of recovery. Patients often feel overwhelmed by the impact of their diagnosis and the physical toll of treatment. Many women find that joining a support group is helpful. Talking with a counselor Or relying on loved ones to help manage mental and emotional stress. It is important to keep in regular contact with your medical professional to manage side effects and adjust your treatment plan if necessary.

Although treatment for ovarian cancer can have serious short-term side effects, But patients are better able to manage their symptoms. Understand the treatment process and get through this difficult time The two main treatments are chemotherapy and surgery. But for patients with BRCA PARP mutations, inhibitors offer a promising add-on. Maintaining remission can help patients who receive appropriate support and care. It is possible to manage side effects and fight for health and well-being during and after treatment.

Coping with long-term side effects

Short-term side effects are often long-term side effects. For example, chemotherapy can have long-term effects. Sometimes peripheral neuropathy cannot be cured. And it can take up to a year for the bladder and bowels to return to normal.

Treatment for ovarian cancer can have long-term side effects that can be just as difficult to manage. with short-term side effects Short-term side effects of chemotherapy and surgery, such as nausea, fatigue, and hair loss, usually go away when treatment ends. But long-term effects can last for months or even years. It must be continuously monitored and adjusted... To better understand the relationship between short-term and long-term side effects The overall treatment process should be taken into account. Patients often experience serious short-term side effects from chemotherapy. Including extreme fatigue, nausea, vomiting, and hair loss, these are outward manifestations of how the body responds to drugs to kill cancer cells. However, long-term side effects usually occur after treatment is complete. And it may not always be immediately clear. But it may have long-term effects on the patient's physical and mental health...

For example, chemotherapy can result in short-term fatigue during treatment. but also long-term chronic fatigue after treatment ends. Some women may experience fatigue several months after completing chemotherapy. Chronic fatigue can interfere with daily activities such as social interaction, employment, and normal movement. It may be more severe than the temporary fatigue that comes with treatment. This may make recovery more challenging and your rest will not improve. By understanding this progress From temporary fatigue to constant fatigue. Patients can prepare for obstacles that may arise during their recovery...

Effects on fertility are another important long-term side effect. Permanent infertility can be caused by chemotherapy and surgery to remove the fallopian tubes or ovaries. As time passes Many women experience feelings of loss or grief. Although the emotional impact of infertility may not be so obvious, Physical changes occur, such as hormonal imbalances that can result in symptoms such as hot flashes or irregular menstrual cycles. These feelings can be intensified as women get used to the new reality of life without being able to conceive… But the emotional impact can occur. More deeply...

Another long-term consequence of chemotherapy is neuropathy, or nerve damage. Many patients experience tingling or numbness in their fingers or toes during treatment. But some people continue to feel this way long after chemotherapy ends. This chronic neuropathy can make daily activities like walking and typing challenging. Chemotherapy can have short-term physical side effects. But the nerve damage remains. Requires rehabilitation or the use of a mobility device. The psychological effects of cancer treatment are another. Short-term emotional distress is common during the initial diagnosis and treatment process. due to side effects Fear of the unknown and the aggressiveness of the treatment. however Emotional scars can last longer than the conclusion of treatment. Chronic emotional problems such as depression or post-traumatic stress disorder can result from concerns about recurrence or physical changes caused by treatment, such as surgical scars. or altered body image as a result of hair loss and need to be taken care of

Changes in blood cell counts can have long-term side effects for women who test positive for BRCA mutations and are treated with PARP inhibitors after chemotherapy. These changes increase your risk of infection or anemia. These side effects Although this is less than the immediate effects of continued chemotherapy. But it can also be permanent and sometimes unpredictable. Additionally, patients may find it more difficult to regain strength because the physical fatigue caused by chronic PARP inhibitor use is superimposed on the pain. Chronic fatigue after chemotherapy.

There is considerable overlap between short-term and long-term side effects. For example, fatigue caused by chemotherapy can last for months and develop into a chronic condition. In the same way Emotional stress after treatment often develops into more chronic psychological problems, such as anxiety, depression, or post-traumatic stress disorder (PTSD). Patients must understand this relationship when advising recovery. Because early symptoms can serve as warning signs of ongoing difficulties…

Managing these long-term side effects requires a comprehensive strategy. Including emotional and physical healing. Patients should cooperate closely with their health care provider to manage ongoing fatigue. nerve damage or mental distress in managing chronic conditions This may include ongoing physical therapy. Consulting nutritional support and in some situations, the use of drugs

Adjusting to a new normal is key to managing the long-term side effects of ovarian cancer treatment. The journey doesn't end when treatment ends. Although immediate side effects may disappear over time. Planning for long-term recovery is easier for patients and their health care teams. When they realize the long-term effects cancer treatment can have on the body and mind A support network to help patients cope with these ongoing difficulties. Whether they come from a family Consulting support group or medical professionals All are necessary things. Patients will feel more empowered to receive the care they need. and work towards a satisfying life after cancer if they understand that these long-term side effects are an extension of the journey to cure.

A short story about Juliana

Juliana is a woman who always succeeds in her daily routine. At the age of forty-two She has created a life that she is proud of. Whether architecture is successful A lovely and loving home All certified families She and her husband of eighteen years, Marcus, raised their daughter, Mia, to be a happy and curious young woman, despite life's hardships. But it felt stable, rooted, and full of hope.

That is, until everything changed in one moment..

It started with a slight stomach ache that she had never known before. At first she didn't care. Thinking it was just the stress of a hard work week, however, the pain continued. Fatigue and bloating soon followed. Problems arose, and Juliana finally saw her doctor a few weeks later. Hoping for a simple explanation But blood tests, scans and tests all pointed to the worst news she could hope for.

Her doctor said softly, "Ovarian cancer," the cold, sharp words still lingering in the air. Third step She felt a shock like she had been kicked in the stomach. Not only was she terrified of the diagnosis; But it also includes intense uncertainty. Ovarian cancer called The "silent killer" has begun to spread. Suddenly her world, her meticulously planned life, would collapse.

The following weeks were filled with endless decisions. Additional testing and counseling Juliana experiences emotions such as anger, denial, disbelief, and fear that are intense and overwhelming. The treatment approach is aggressive. Surgery to remove as much of the tumor as possible Chemotherapy is then used to eliminate any remaining cancer cells. Nothing could prepare her for the reality of the side effects. Even though she had heard about it.
above all else Had surgery which was successful. But Juliana felt empty. Her body was weak and intense sadness came in a quiet moment when she realized how much her body had changed. And although the scar is a constant reminder of the battle she is facing, But it was the chemotherapy that changed her.

The dizziness from the first chemotherapy hit her hard. She couldn't identify herself in the mirror. Her face locked. Pale and glistening with sweat She felt more exposed and vulnerable as her hair began to fall out and her head was shaved. He will be on his stomach. Some days she was too weak to care for Mia or stay long enough to eat. And she could barely move the bed. She felt like her body, mind, and soul were all alien.

But the biggest impact on her was loneliness. Cancer treatment is isolating, every day feels like a struggle. And even though he loves and supports But Marcus couldn't fully understand her struggle. Juliana misses being a strong, confident woman. It is the pillar of support for her family. She felt herself disappear. Becoming a shadow of the person she used to be

But there was a short period. As well, her family's love carried her through difficult times. Marcus was always by her side. He comforted her when she felt overwhelmed and held her hand every time she gave medicine, even though Mia was too young to fully understand the gravity of the situation. But she still makes her mother laugh and smile with her silly antics. Juliana finds herself clinging to memories of better days. When everything seems easy and satisfying.

Side effects become more bearable as chemotherapy progresses. Fatigue never goes away. But her body began to adjust. Some days she struggles to get out of bed. But some days she can get up and walk. Even if it's just a small thing Around the building and a glimmer of hope appeared as soft strands of hair sprouted behind it.

However, it is never easy. There were days when she wanted to quit because she was so depressed. She was constantly afraid of a recurrence. And the healing seems to last forever. She spent many restless nights thinking about her future. What happens if the cancer returns? What if treatment is not enough? It was a quiet, melancholy moment that almost destroyed her.

One afternoon, Juliana was sitting on the couch, covered in a blanket, in what looked like her 100th chemotherapy session. Juliana had never seen Mia playing nearby. The thought of surviving and facing this disease with courage consumed her thoughts. She tried to concentrate on the here and now. But the weight of the future hung heavy. Make her hands shake

Then Mia's innocent voice pierced Juliana's thoughts as she looked up at her doll.

The question is simple. But it hit Juliana like a wave. Tears welled in her eyes as she struggled to answer. How can she promise Mia forever? How could she promise something she didn't know?

"You will always be the best, right Mom?"

Despite the pain, Juliana said with a gentle smile, "I don't know if I'll be good forever, darling." "But I'm trying, I promise."

And in that moment something changed. It was a quiet realization rather than a big reveal. She doesn't need to know everything. She doesn't have to make a lifelong commitment. The important thing is that you continue to love, fight, and try. For Mia's sake For Marcus' sake for his own benefit

Juliana learned to embrace uncertainty and not let it overwhelm her as the months passed. Her cancer is in remission. Her strength gradually returned, and her hair grew longer again. Even though they still felt like they were chained. But the physical scars were gone. Juliana discovered a new sense of purpose and gratitude in life. she is happy every day laugh with friends Holding Marcus' hand And watch Mia grow. One evening a year Juliana stood in her garden. Her hair blows gently in the breeze. It is a bright and cute flower. And the flowers you planted are in full bloom. Marcus stepped closer and stood beside her. With his arm around her shoulders
"You look better," he said, his voice full of pride and love.

Juliana smiled and said. "I feel better." Even a small smile is sincere, because it came through hardships, tears, and small victories. And when the sun begins to set Juliana suddenly realized something important. Cancer doesn't take away the love of her life, her family, and her soul. It made her stronger despite her failed attempts. The light of a new beginning Filled with laughter, hope, and the hope that the days will last longer. has replaced the storm

In addition to surviving cancer Juliana also rediscovers happiness. and finally Hers is her greatest victory.

Part 7

Addressing the mental challenge on ovarian cancer

Living with the long-term effects of ovarian cancer can be emotionally and mentally taxing. This is because it may include the period immediately after treatment. and adjustment to later life after ovarian cancer management or remission. A person's emotional state can change as a result of treatment, recovery, and prolonged uncertainty about the future. And these difficulties can change at any time.

The main mental health issues that people with ovarian cancer have to deal with are depression, anxiety and fear. These feelings are not just related to cancer. But it also includes treatment approaches and results. This is because ovarian cancer is often discovered at an advanced stage. This can make the patient feel weak. Fear of recurrence is therefore a major obstacle. And uncertainty about whether the cancer will return can lead to constant underwater stress. This fear may manifest as anxiety. As a result, people are hyper-aware of their bodies and any changes to them. that may occur This may make them feel even more stressed. the need to "Living in the present" becomes an internal struggle as a result of constant fear of the future.

Physical changes caused by the disease and its treatment can also cause anxiety. Hormonal Imbalance Weight changes, hair loss, and fatigue are just some of the side effects that can result from chemotherapy, surgery, and radiation. These physical changes can affect a person's self-worth and image. Because many People struggle with the way they view themselves and the way they believe others view them. These changes can therefore have significant psychological consequences. It can lead to feelings of social isolation or loneliness and shame. Failure to perform duties or maintain responsibilities (such as being a carer or employee) can have a negative impact on one's sense of self. and may result in deterioration of mental health...

Additionally, when patients are dealing with the difficulty of managing chronic health problems. Their emotional flexibility is often tested. The anticipatory cycle of anxiety can be stimulated by constant check-ups and testing. which can trigger feelings of fear Feelings of helplessness or lack of control may result from the need for constant monitoring and the possibility of additional intervention or procedures. Managing the emotional and physical stress of ovarian cancer can be exhausting. and aggravate mental health problems

Another common problem for cancer survivors is mental fatigue. Balancing treatment plans doctor appointments And emotional stress can be very difficult. These constant demands tend to become emotionally exhausting over time. People feel tired or lack the energy to have healthy relationships or do the things that used to make them happy. This feeling of apathy and withdrawal caused by fatigue can worsen depression.
Social support is important in dealing with these mental health issues. But they are often complex and constantly changing. Friends and family may not always understand the intensity of feelings of loneliness resulting from the emotional damage caused by cancer. Especially when they don't want to burden the people they love. And it can be challenging for many people to communicate feelings of fear and uncertainty. The difficulty here is not only providing the physical support needed, but But it also demonstrates the emotional understanding and compassion needed to validate a survivor's experience. People may feel less alone in their journey if they find others who truly understand, such as a support group or other cancer survivors.

Ovarian cancer also affects emotional relationships. Intimacy problems can occur in couples. This is especially true if the other person feels less safe or physically detached. Some people experience increased emotional stress when they think of losing their fertility or being unable to conceive after treatment. The strain on relationships caused by these personal problems increases the mental difficulties of living with cancer.

Living with the long-term effects of ovarian cancer requires adapting to an ever-changing world. Therapists and counselors are examples of mental health professionals who play an important role in supporting cancer survivors as they process their emotions and develop coping mechanisms for anxiety. Depression and fear: Stress reduction and mindfulness practices, such as yoga or meditation. It can be a helpful resource to help people reconnect with their bodies. and reduce mental stress. For some people, engaging in support or finding meaning in their experiences can give them a sense of direction and Reduce their helplessness

Addressing the mental health issues related to ovarian cancer requires a comprehensive strategy. This includes self-compassion. Social interaction, therapy, and emotional support It acknowledges the complex emotional and psychological burdens that persist long after treatment. People can cope with mental and emotional stress. and get the help they need to build coping mechanisms that will improve their quality of life...

Educating the future generation

An important first step in increasing early detection and help create effective treatment is to educate the next generation about ovarian cancer and its importance. Although ovarian cancer receives less attention than other types of cancer, But the impact is great. And educating is more important than ever. In addition to raising public awareness about the disease, The aim is to educate young people on how to recognize potential warning signs. The value of health screening and how to promote a supportive and compassionate environment for those affected.

Educating the next generation about the symptoms and risk factors for ovarian cancer is one of the first steps. of providing knowledge about ovarian cancer Symptoms of ovarian cancer are different from other types of cancer. Often vague and easily confused with symptoms of other medical conditions, these symptoms, which are often mistaken for less severe medical conditions, include bloating, pain in the lower abdomen or stomach. Difficulty eating and frequent urination Early detection It is important to increase survival rates. And teach young people about these symptoms and, if they persist, it is worth getting medical help. and learning to detect early It may occur when ovarian cancer is detected early. As people become more aware of this disease The more effective your treatment options will be.

In addition to being aware of the symptoms of ovarian cancer, Educating the next generation about risk factors is important Important risk factors include inherited gene mutations, such as BRCA1 and BRCA2, and genetic factors, such as family history of ovarian cancer, breast cancer, and other cancers. Educating young people about the availability of genetic testing and the part of genetics in ovarian cancer is important. Being aware of these risk factors allows people to take preventive measures, such as closely monitoring their health. and seek genetic counseling if necessary. This is because they have more control over their own health decisions. It also helps them feel less afraid or uncertain.

Another important component of the study is to inform future generations about ovarian cancer prevention strategies and research advances. Lifestyle changes and certain preventive measures can reduce your risk of ovarian cancer. Although there is no way to avoid it. Educating young people about healthy lifestyle choices, such as quitting smoking Maintaining a balanced diet And regular exercise can greatly help prevent cancer. Additionally, teaching young people about research advances, such as the promise of new treatments and methods for early detection, can promote a worldview in Optimism and support for cancer research projects Awareness of progress may encourage them to seek clinical trials or become involved in health advocacy.

Focusing on developing a culture of compassion and support for individuals affected by ovarian cancer is equally important. Cancer has a huge mental and emotional impact. which is often overlooked We can cultivate empathy by teaching young people to support friends, family, or classmates who have been diagnosed with ovarian cancer. This includes recognizing the special difficulties faced by cancer patients, such as adverse drug reactions. mental stress and anxiety of recurrence We can guarantee a more encouraging environment. Where those affected by the disease feel understood and validated by teaching young people to consider the needs of cancer.

Potential stigma and misunderstandings surrounding this disease This must also be addressed in ovarian cancer education. Honest conversations about women's health issues in general are lacking. And many people ignore the difficulties faced by women with ovarian cancer. We can overcome these barriers by integrating conversations about ovarian cancer into public health initiatives and school curricula. A society that is more informed and less critical of health issues may result in promoting discussion about women's health. cancer prevention and personal well-being Ensuring we know the importance of supporting those affected by ovarian cancer...

Reaching young people and having meaningful conversations with them about ovarian cancer can be done in many ways in the digital age. Educational videos Interactive campaigns And social media is a powerful tool for raising awareness. Enabling young people to educate friends and family about ovarian cancer has the potential to spread knowledge and change attitudes. Universities and schools can participate. An important part of integrating cancer awareness initiatives into the health education curriculum. To allow students to learn about ovarian cancer and other general cancer prevention topics.

In the end Educating the next generation about ovarian cancer goes beyond just providing information. That includes promoting support, empathy and a sense of duty. Encouraging young people to identify warning signs and symptoms of ovarian cancer. Understand risk factors and speak on behalf of those affected by this disease It is equally important to normalize honest conversations about women's health and cancer. and create a culture of understanding and support. By using this comprehensive educational approach We can therefore ensure that the next generation is better equipped to deal with the hardships posed by ovarian cancer. Support awareness campaigns and ultimately help people with this serious disease achieve better outcomes.

Conclusion

Ovarian Cancer: Breaking the Silence and Raising Awareness for Women and Young People serves as a call to action. It is as well a powerful reminder of our collective responsibility to help create a future where ovarian cancer is recognized, understood and treated with compassion and urgency. Ovarian cancer has been hidden for too long due to a lack of knowledge. Misunderstandings about symptoms and the stigma often associated with women's health concerns. And this book attempts to end that silence by emphasizing the importance of early detection. giving knowledge and support We must not allow this disease to go unnoticed by ensuring that future generations of women and men are protected. Go understand the risks, recognize the signs and actively participate in a culture of prevention and care.

In addition to educating women and youth on recognizing early warning signs, Increasing their awareness also gives them the confidence to speak up about their own health and wellbeing. Women should be empowered to trust their instincts, ask questions and seek medical advice when symptoms arise. Due to early detection of ovarian cancer It remains the most effective way to increase survival from ovarian cancer. Understanding the disease and preventing its spread depends heavily on education about genetic and environmental risk factors. A society where all women feel informed and supported is more likely to succeed when we normalize discussions about ovarian cancer.

Ending the taboo around ovarian cancer also means strengthening empathy and ensuring that those affected don't just have to deal with their own suffering. By creating an environment that values honest communication. We enable women to talk about their struggles, successes, and experiences without fear of criticism or misinterpretation. This sense of belonging is important to the advancement of ovarian cancer research and treatment as well as emotional healing. The more we give voice to those affected, The more we spread the word that their experiences matter. And their opinions will play a key role in shaping future cancer treatments.

We must look to the future and push new research. and further advances in the treatment of ovarian cancer At the same time, they emphasize the importance of early detection. and preventive care This includes promoting screening procedures for high-risk individuals. Expand access to genetic counseling Push for more funding for research We need to make sure the next generation knows they can make a difference in the fight against ovarian cancer. They can actively participate by participating in support campaigns. Provide funding for cancer research And above all, spreading the word about awareness. We finally have the potential to change the perception of ovarian cancer. By empowering women and youth and educating them about it. Together, we will make ovarian cancer a disease we understand, fight, and overcome. Instead of being a silent killer We can promote early detection. successful treatment and finally, treatment through sustainable awareness campaigns. Healthcare initiatives and people's personal dedication to supporting their own health. This book is just the beginning as no one else has to face ovarian cancer. This is thanks to a wide-ranging movement that defies taboos. Raise awareness and demonstrates the power of a united community. By working together Can we reverse this trend? and provide a healthy and informed future for future generations.

Reference

https://www.dovepress.com/identification-of-differentially-expressed-genes-and-signaling-pathway-peer-reviewed-article-OTT

Overview: The WHO's Health for All initiative, launched in 1977, aims to ensure universal access to healthcare and improve the quality of life for people worldwide.

National Cancer Institute – Ovarian Cancer (PDQ®)

- National Cancer Institute - Ovarian Cancer
- **Overview**: This resource from the U.S. National Cancer Institute offers detailed information about ovarian cancer, including research on its causes, risk factors, and the latest advancements in treatment and prevention. The PDQ cancer database is regularly updated with current research findings.

American Cancer Society – Ovarian Cancer Overview

- **Link**: American Cancer Society - Ovarian Cancer
- **Overview**: The American Cancer Society provides a comprehensive overview of ovarian cancer, including its risk factors, symptoms, stages, diagnosis, and treatment options. This resource is widely regarded as a trusted source for understanding various cancers.

Ovarian Cancer Research Alliance (OCRA)

- **Link**: OCRA
- **Overview**: OCRA is a leading organization dedicated to funding research on ovarian cancer and providing support to those affected by it. Their website offers both patient-centered information and insights into the latest ovarian cancer research.

www.ingramcontent.com/pod-product-compliance
Lightning Source LLC
Chambersburg PA
CBHW071108240526
45469CB00006BD/2391